secret a long life

Life up to 120 years
Hunza tribes and blue zones

IDET BY: D.SALADIN
Publisher :Yazan and Loay Press and Publishing

ISBN: 9781792846885

only eat to live

index

Introduction

At the point when researchers found the "blue zones" a couple of years prior—four confined geographic zones where individuals were living past the age of 100 at up to multiple times the ordinary rate—they thought about whether they may have discovered the underpinnings of the wellspring of youth. Clearly the DNA of these centenarians, or their way of life, or their sustenance sources, held responses for every one of us.

Since the logical papers have been distributed and the display blurred, solemn news is developing. It appears that a portion of these little pockets of life span are ceasing to exist, as the more up to date ages' Western-impacted way of life and diet converts into poorer wellbeing and lower future.

In 2000, Michel Poulain, a Belgian demographer, had recently completed the process of affirming, one by one, the time of centenarians in Sardinia, Italy, when he understood that "these centenarians are gathered in one zone." He snatched a brilliant turquoise blue marker and orbited the towns where he'd discovered centenarians, actually putting the primary "blue zone" on a guide.

He has since progressed toward becoming, in his own words, "the underwriter of the legitimacy of life span," venturing to the far corners of the planet to discover and logically approve life span zones. He needs solid records to check that each centenarian is really 100 years of age or more. He at that point ascertains the centenarian rate, estimating their focus in a geographic territory: one Sardinian town of 3,000 individuals had 42 centenarians in the previous 30 years, he says, though the normal Belgian town of a similar size had "possibly one."".

Blue areas were not observed until 2005, with exploratory missions reaching the areas already known to scientists, as well as in Okinawa, Japan and Sardinia, as "blue zones."

Older people in blue areas not only live longer, they also reach old age in great mental and physical health. However.,

They had simple pleasures: a midday nap and social work every day. The lifestyle that maintained health in old age was shaped by their living conditions - which applied to all four blue areas. Their environment was improved through longevity.

But now the inhabitants of the Blue Zone are no longer living in isolation from the rest of the world.

Some blue areas are more resistant to change. In Nicoya.

Secrets of a long life

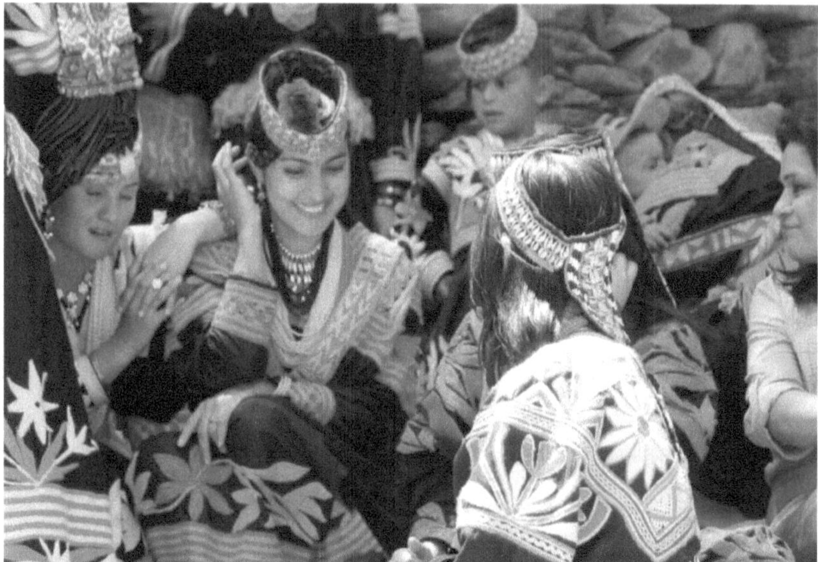

We may not know, and after extensive studies and research, we found that eating habits and the area in which people live have a relationship to longevity and long happy life,

Hunza tribes do not know diseases or aging.

Cancer does not know women who give birth at the age of 60 and breed men in the 1990s as if they were from another planet

Average age is 120 years

how is that possible? How do they stay healthy? What are their secrets? Let us know these secrets

And how scientists were able to study the dietary habits of these tribes,

Which were found to be similar to those of people living in blue areas

In this book, we will know the secret of their long lives and what they eat and drink

Life Expectancy

The HONZA rate is 120 years

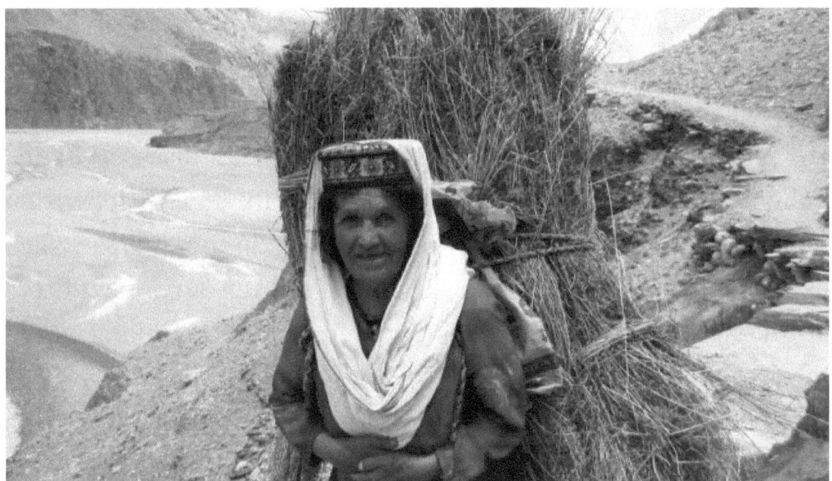

There are no chemicals or additives in their diet.

It is very common for a Hunzas woman to have children after the age of 60.

It may seem shocking to you, but Hunzas can be ready.

The crew are discovered by the locals and brought to a quiet valley where they find refuge from the storm. The citizens of this magical place are said to be hundreds of years old, devoid of disease and excellent health. A sick member of the convoy begins to regain strength, while the age of each individual appears to be suspended in time. When you leave anyone from the Shangri-La characters, they return to their real age.

It is wonderful that the Hunza tribes, as well as their age of not less than one hundred and up to one hundred and twenty, but many of them up to one hundred and sixty are not nearly and do not suffer from health problems or chronic diseases or diseases of children suffered by all the peoples of the world has not registered for hundreds of years Any of these diseases for any citizen has an understanding does not get cancer, appendicitis, gastric ulcers, tension, anxiety or fatigue and does not suffer from diseases of the colon and no problems in the abdomen and nerves and do not suffer from any problems such as diseases of the yellow or kidney stones or bones or heart and hypertension Blood, diabetes and obesity. Many diseases in urban areas, such as poliomyelitis and measles, have never been recorded. There are no special needs cases, and women still have children up to the age of 65.

How to combat aging

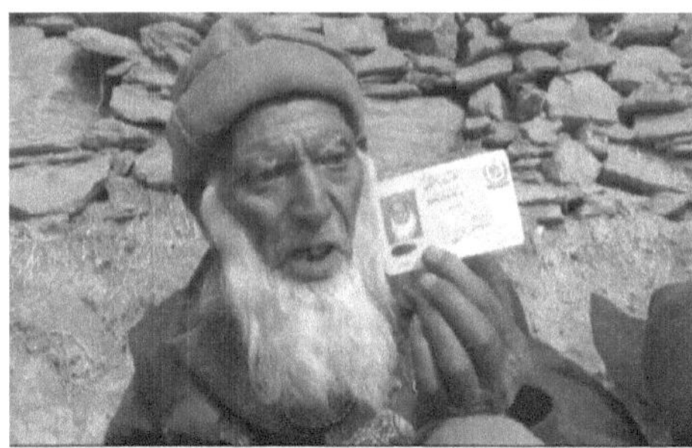

and physical deterioration and enjoy health and happiness People living in blue areas share common lifestyle characteristics that contribute to their longevity. The Venn scheme on the right highlights the following six common characteristics among the inhabitants of Okinawa, Sardinia

Mohammed - raise other concerns

Less smoking

Semi-vegetarian - Most of the food consumed is derived from plants

Constant moderate physical activity - an integral part of life

Social participation - people of all ages are socially active and integrated into their communities

Legumes - usually consumed

lifestyle of people in blue zones:

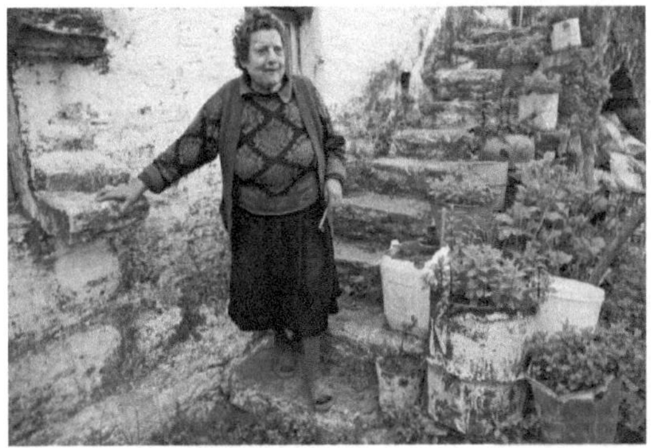

Moderate, regular physical activity.
Life purpose.
Stress reduction.
Moderate caloric intake.
Plant-based diet.
Moderate alcohol intake, especially wine.
Engagement in spirituality or religion.
Engagement in family life.
Engagement in social life

These blue areas share one point, which is characterized by sunny, well-ventilated areas. It is also characterized by different food systems but at the same time have two sides in common. The first is to rely on plants to feed on meat, fish and cheese only during occasions or in small quantities. The second is their eating of vegetables. At the taste level, the diets vary greatly from region to region. If the inhabitants of Ikaria have a diet close to the Mediterranean diet (vegetables, olive oil, legumes, fruits, whole grains, fish and white meat), the inhabitants of the mountain villages of Sardinia do not consume fish but meat

Mobility and movement is a key factor in prolonging the lives of these areas, where they remain active and in more natural ways, such as gardening, grazing, walking, cycling, etc. Interest in the faith is the other one of the most important factors that make the elderly in a good psychological and spiritual, which have lower levels of depression and cardiovascular disease, the cause of the first death.

In addition to the above, there is the family bonding factor, which is a priority for the inhabitants of the blue areas, as charity and care seem to ultimately lead to more happiness, and push people towards a healthy lifestyle.

Several studies have confirmed that vegetables and fruits are powerful weapons to fight aging and preserve young people's taste, because they are foods rich in antioxidant flavonoids and carotenoids.

Dr. Oz has identified a range of foods that are resistant to signs of aging and limit their appearance at an early age.

Mulberry

One of the most important types of antioxidant fruit, it is recommended to eat one unit a day on a regular basis.

Beans

Beans contain a high protein content that helps nourish and strengthen hair follicles.

Cranberry juice

The berries protect the teeth from yellowing, as well as its role in the fight against bacteria causing decay, but doctors advise to eat without sugar.

Bloody orange

Orange is the blood of citrus rich in anthocyanin and antioxidants, which helps to combat aging.

Islands

Of vegetables very rich in vitamin A, which plays a key role in maintaining the scalp and adds to the hair shine.

Nuts

The nuts contain selenium, which helps to renew cells and protect them from aging, as well as their role in burning harmful fats, so doctors advise to eat two units of nuts daily on a regular basis.

Dark chocolate

Very rich in antioxidant flavonoids also.

Red wine

Red wines are made from grape seeds rich in antioxidant polyphenols. Doctors for non-drinkers can add resveratrol in pharmacies to grape juice to play the same role.

cod

Contains an abundant amount of anti-aging selenium, which keeps the skin from harmful sun rays and protects against cancer.

Low-fat cheese

Contains important proteins for the body especially hair follicles.

Option

One of the most useful vegetables for the skin, because it contains the «silica» that resist the emergence of wrinkles, as it works to increase collagen in the skin.

Kelp

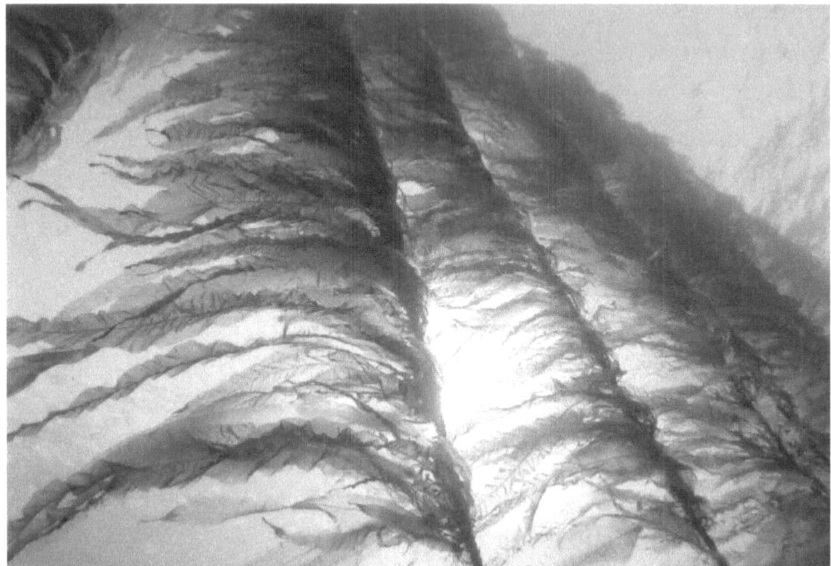

It is a plant that grows in the sea and contains vitamin C and E, so it helps to maintain skin fat, which prevents the appearance of wrinkles early.

Eggs

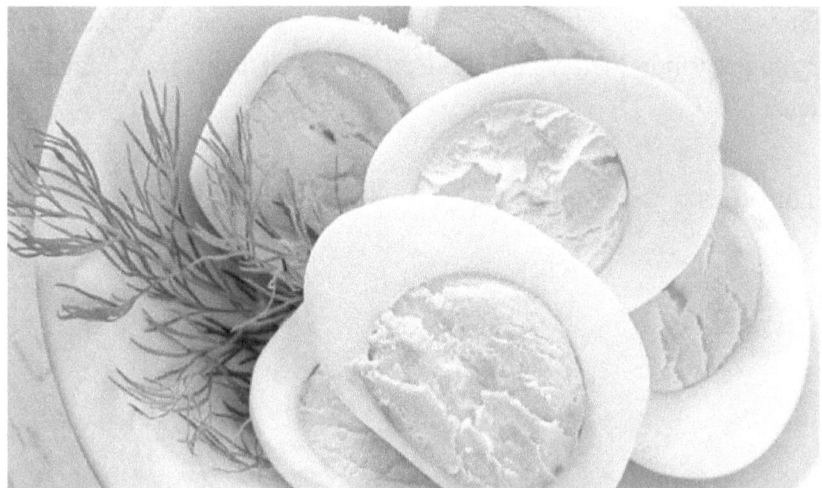

Eggs are a favorite breakfast for many, and doctors have confirmed that containing iron and protein makes it a good food for skin and hair.

Guava

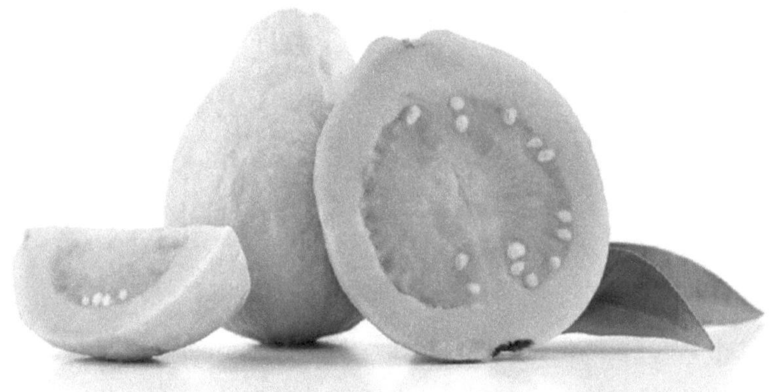

Guava contains vitamin C, which promotes the production of collagen, and doctors are advised to eat at least two guavas a week.

Tomatoes

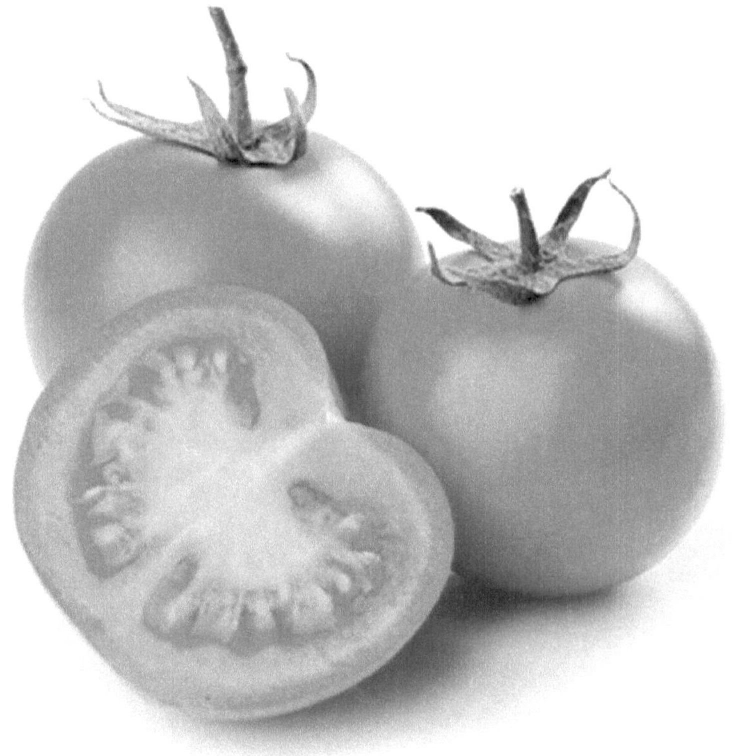

Rich in lycopene that resists heart disease, cancer and cholesterol, as well as its role as harmful sun rays that may cause skin dryness and dark spots.

Beef

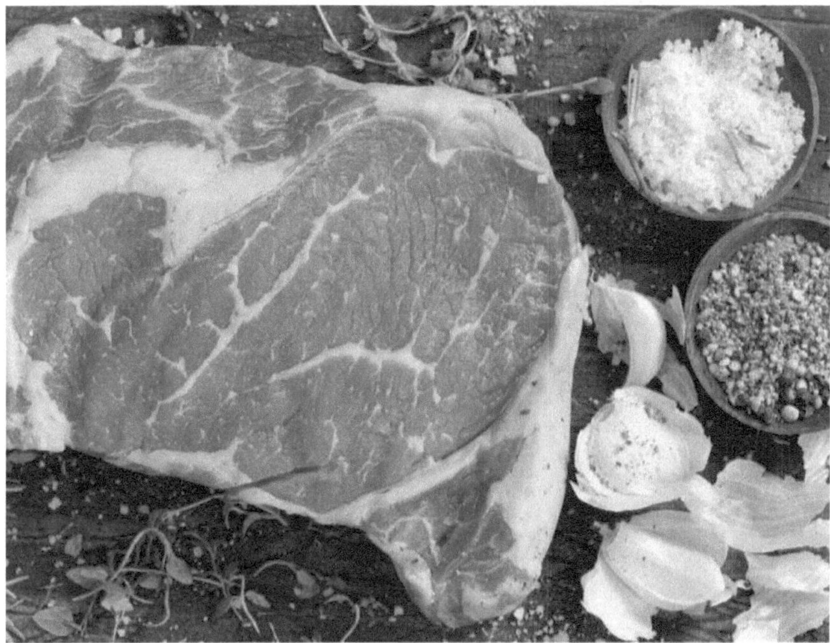

Small beef is especially rich in iron which plays an important role in maintaining nails.

Did you know that there are healthy foods that resist disease and aging and give you a happy life? Yes, it is confirmed by the fact d. Elizabeth Super is the author of several books on healthy nutrition, explaining that good food avoids taking medicine and resisting physical and mental deterioration, so you are offered a package of foods that strengthen your body and help it to resist

diseases.

To combat stress, take the seeds of sunflower "Syrian pulp" because it is a good source of folic acid, which helps the brain to produce a chemistry called "Duamein", which achieve happiness, eat a small amount of it between meals.

Studies have shown that magnesium found in green leaves such as spinach improves the body's resistance to stress. Try eating it on the day when you feel irritable and tense and add it to the salad to increase its nutritional value.

- Charge your body by eating almonds, which helps to stabilize the level of energy in the body thanks to the mixture of protein and healthy fats that contain so try a small amount of it with a slice of apples or a biscuit and use this snack to provide energy in the middle of the day.

 - Eat an egg or two eggs at breakfast with a slice of brown bread from whole wheat to get a basic meal provides you with energy and vitality and fight fatigue.

- Eat the insomnia by eating skimmed yogurt. Calcium-rich foods increase the level of serotonin, the hormone that sleeps. Take a cup of skimmed milk two hours before bedtime. Bananas contain vitamin B6, which helps regulate sleep hours so be sure to eat one fruit a day Also potatoes, which studies have proven to be a drug that affects the drug. If you suffer from insomnia, eat half of the potato fruit before going to sleep four hours.

- To keep your memory sharp, eat salmon and omega-3 fatty acids can reduce the risk of infections, which reduces the risk of mental illness, as well as olive oil. Studies have shown that those who rely on food to cook this oil less susceptible to Alzheimer's disease So be sure to take two tablespoons of it daily.

- Studies at Harvard University have shown that women who eat a small piece of cheese or whole-fat dairy products are more fertile than those who do not. They eat a piece of cheese a day, and the lentils that are given in this study are as important With regard to its positive impact on the fertility of women, where it was proved that women who abstained from eating animal proteins and replace lentils increased the chance of giving them by 50% try eating a meal rich in vegetable protein instead of animal and I want to eat Ain Jamal and its useful color to Fertility Aadh.

- Burn fat by eating chili because it contains calcium, which increases the metabolism and consumption of soybeans and products because the studies conducted at the University of Illinois showed that soy milk helps the body to control the proportion of fat in it, as well as green tea to burn fat and increase the speed of metabolism and to know On the chili pepper

- Stimulate your immune system by taking cantaloupe. One cup gives you more than 100% of your daily needs of vitamin C. Eat it several times a week. Broccoli also contains antioxidant-rich vegetables that fight hot, pathogenic and inflammatory bacteria.

Take it several times a week. Rich in zinc and minerals that help your body fight disease.

- Headaches struggled with cowpea, where studies have shown that the instability of the level of sugar in the blood is what leads to suffering in headaches and eat cowpea rich in protein and fiber occurs balance in sugar and protects you from headaches and eating tuna containing Omega 3, which inhibits infections leading to migraines.

Finally, to maintain your skin tone and softness, the expert recommends eating black and red berries because it is rich in antioxidants that fight aging

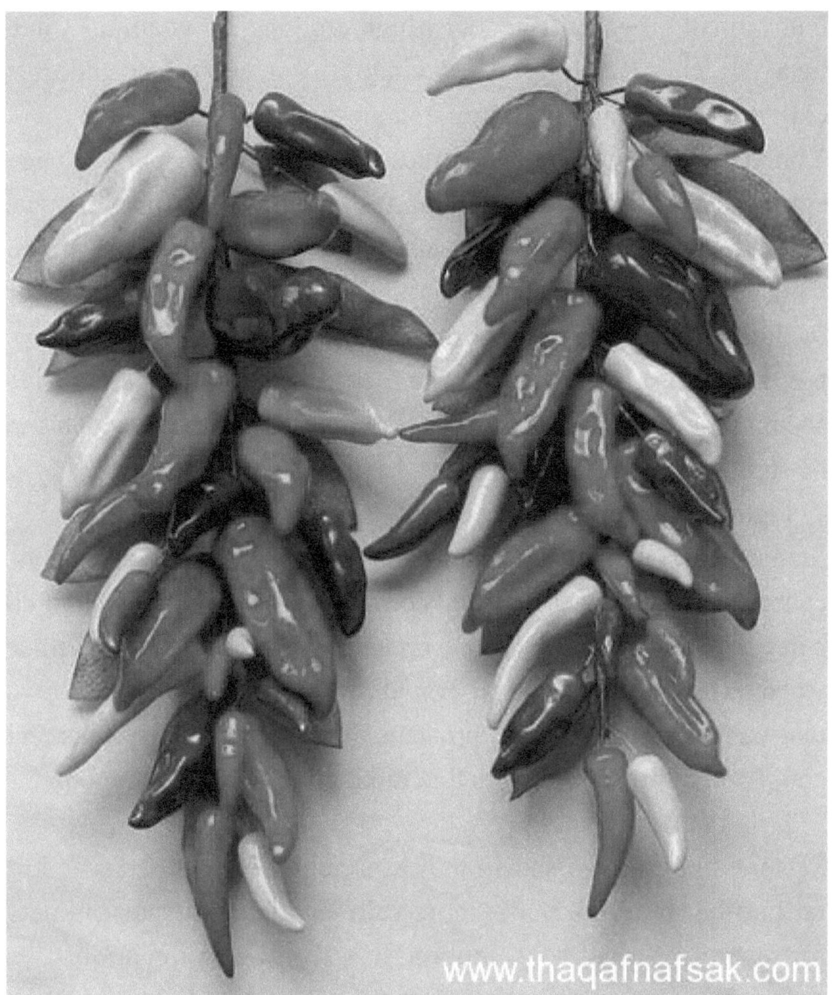

Chili has been in human food since more than 7,500 years BC, and its cultivation was confined to South America until it was discovered by Christopher Columbus and spread throughout the world.

Nutritionally, hot chili contains high amounts of vitamin C, and beta-carotene, which turns into vitamin A as needed. In addition, chili provides vitamins B, iron, magnesium, and potassium.

You may be a person who likes to eat peppers, but they are confused about their effect on human health, where many believe that the flame-burning sensation in peppers causes health damage. In fact, the capsaicin found in chili and responsible for the hot taste of chili pepper has received considerable attention in the scientific community, where research and studies have accumulated that showed its benefits on human health, which can be summarized as follows:

1) Fighting cancerous diseases:

Studies have shown that capsaicin, which is found in peppers, causes prostate cancer cells to "commit suicide". In one study, 80 percent of cancer cells in the prostate were eliminated in mice when exposed to capsaicin. In addition, researchers have shown that cancer tumors in the prostate have shrunk to five percent compared to prostate tumors that did not receive this compound.

2) Helps in weight loss:

Several studies have shown that capsaicin increases the speed of fat burning by 30%, burns more calories and stimulates fullness for several hours of consumption. It is worth mentioning that the consumption of caffeine in coffee or tea after chili increases the effectiveness of capsaicin.

3) Contributes to the treatment of gastrointestinal disorders:

Studies suggest that capsaicin may help eliminate H. pylori, which causes acidity and heartburn, which increases the risk of ulcers and stomach cancer.

On the other hand, studies have shown that consumption of chili does not lead to any damage to the lining of the stomach or intestines, but protects them from bacterial infections.

4) play a role in the prevention and treatment of diabetes:

Researchers in Canada have confirmed that injecting mice with capsaicin helps to cure type 1 diabetes (insulin-dependent). There have been no experiments on humans in this area, and attempts to study the mechanisms are continuing. However, an Australian study found that consumption of hot peppers caused a decrease in levels of insulin and sugar following meals compared to cases where the consumption of chili was not consumed.

The researchers believe that capsaicin improves the body's sensitivity to insulin, which improves sugar balance and reduces the risk of diabetes.

5) Reduces the risk of cardiovascular disease:

Studies have shown that capsaicin may lower the level of cholesterol and triglycerides in the blood as well as plate aggregation. In addition, studies indicate that communities that consume hot chili often have lower rates of cardiovascular disease than those they rarely consume.

6) Reduces the symptoms of migraines:

Capsaicin may help treat migraines because it inhibits the neurotransmitter called P which is responsible for pain. On the other hand, other research studies the role of capsaicin as an effective anesthetic for teeth.

7) Reduces sinus congestion:

Capsaicin stimulates sinus secretions, reducing congestion, and possesses anti-bacterial properties that fight sinus infections

Research confirms that there are many foods that have some anti-aging qualities when taken regularly, and it helps prevent some diseases related to aging also as heart disease, diabetes and osteoporosis, yet foods that anti-aging foods represent a new hope to get rid of complications of aging, So you can follow a healthy and integrated diet while continuing to exercise and it will work to resist aging significantly.

Here are the most important foods that help to resist aging and its symptoms

1 - nuts - nuts

Contains a high proportion of omega-3 fatty acids and essential acids, it also improves the level of cholesterol and improves digestive performance.

2 - berries

Researchers have discovered that berries contain some substances that help to reduce inflammation and avoid oxidative damage.

3- Green plants

Green plants contain calcium, folic acid and some healthy foods that maintain bone health and help to fight eye diseases as they age. These vegetables, such as cabbage and broccoli, also reduce the risk of cancer and loss of memory.

Dark chocolate

Cocoa beans, which produce dark chocolate, as well as antioxidants, flavanol, reduce skin infections caused by exposure to ultraviolet rays, activate blood circulation, improve skin's ability to retain moisture, reduce skin wrinkles and make them appear smaller. Senna.

5. Beans

Studies have shown that beans are the ideal food for the heart and provide a great source of low fat protein, especially for vegetarians. In addition, it is full of fiber, which helps to reduce the cholesterol, and contains vitamins, minerals, antioxidants, potassium, iron and vitamin B.

6. Whole grains

As it contains fibers, minerals, vitamins, antioxidants and vitamin B, and works to reduce the risk of diseases of aging, such as cancer and cardiovascular disease, and because of the slow digestion rate is very useful for the prevention of diabetes and high blood pressure.

Fish

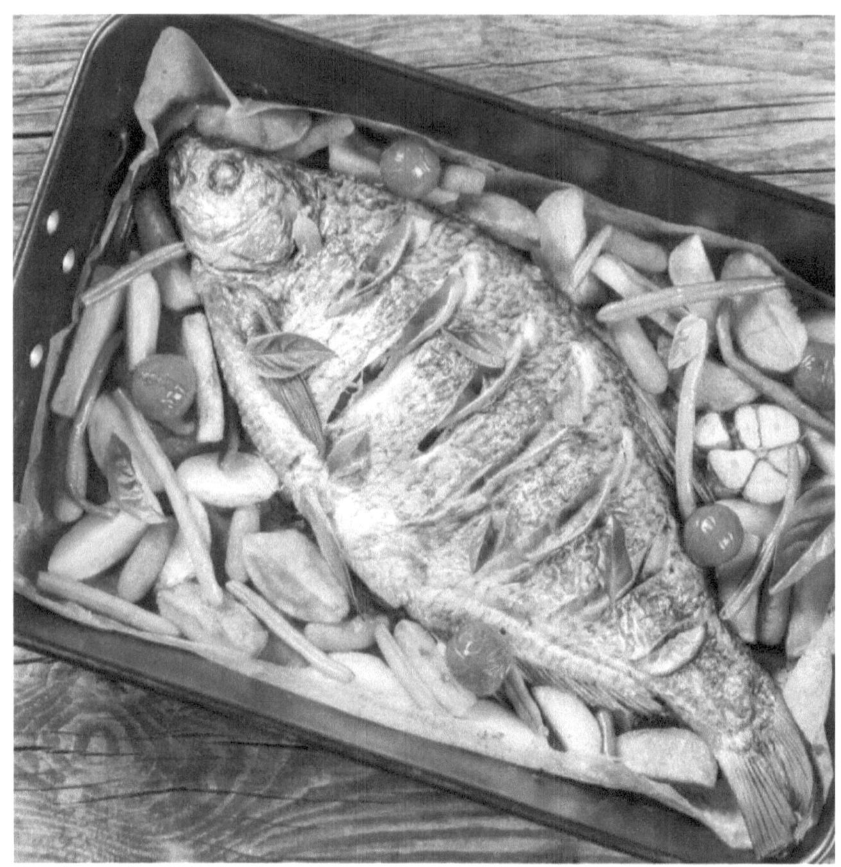

Seafood is rich in important fatty acids such as omega-3, which affects the center of the brain responsible for improving mood, and omega-3 found in tuna and salmon has a strong anti-inflammatory effect.

8. Olive oil

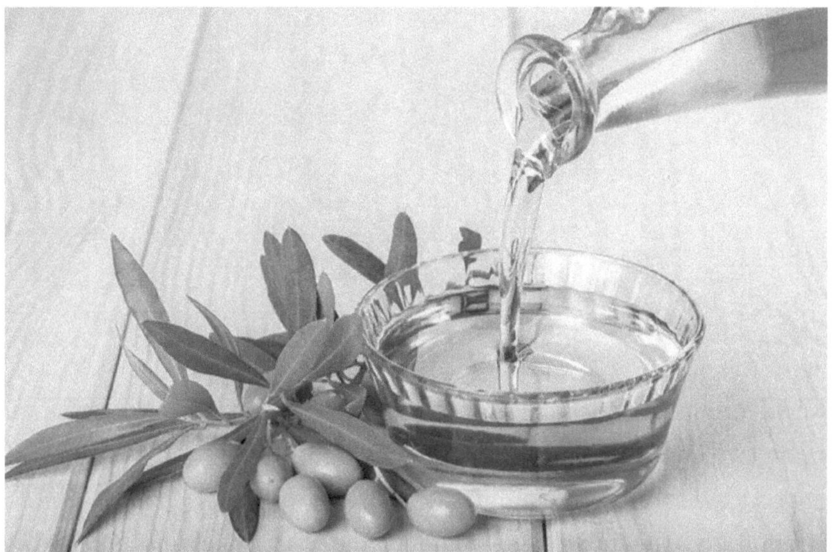

Scientists have recently discovered that olive oil contains large amounts of monounsaturated fats important for the health of the body and heart and resists aging.

9. Kiwi

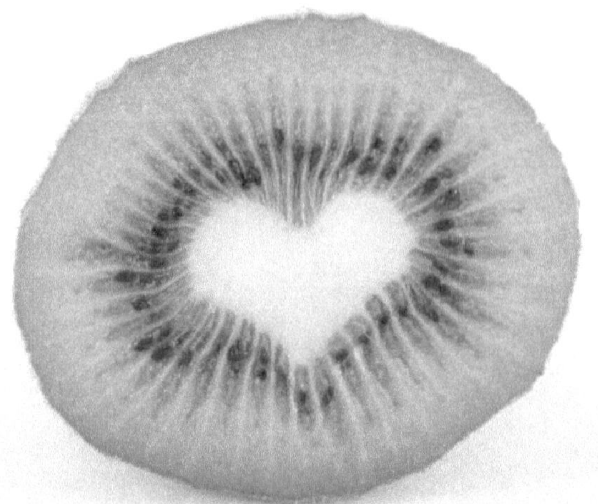

Kiwi contains a high proportion of vitamin C greater than oranges and bananas also contains a high proportion of antioxidants and is a good source of magnesium, which strengthens the heart and protects the blood vessels and helps absorb energy from food.

10. Honey

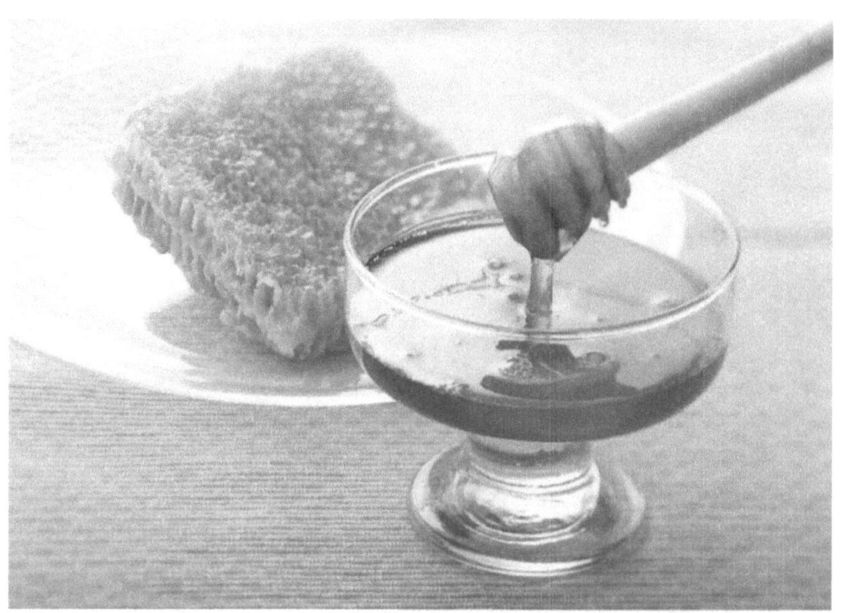

It contains a lot of food, the most important of which is carbohydrates and water. It is considered an effective anti-inflammatory and is also resistant to viruses and colds. In addition, there are many foods that help slow the appearance of aging such as garlic, which helps to reduce cholesterol and blood pressure, and green pepper, which is a great source of vitamin C and promotes the production of collagen important for the health and appearance of the skin, and the islands strengthens the immune system and helps to protect the skin on In addition, soybeans are important and very useful especially for women who have reached menopause to contain a high proportion of is flavones, which helps to reduce bone loss that always occurs in menopause

Foods that fight skin

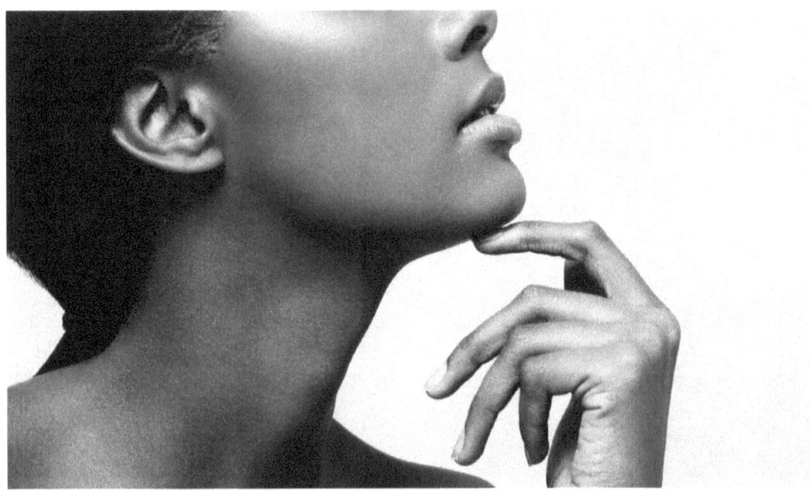

Despite the enormous revolution caused by anti-wrinkle creams and other cosmetic methods such as injections and packaging; but there is a link between the foods we eat daily and the health of the skin, it can hurt the skin and give the opposite effect if we eat the wrong foods, such as increased fat or increased appearance of pimples. Proper nutrition appropriate for skin type can avoid high care and treatment costs.

Women should receive the largest share of their daily diet of fresh fruits and vegetables and grains, as well as meat, milk and dairy products, and reduce the intake of fat, especially if they suffer from the problem of facial pills or skin fats.

There is a list of foods that we consider best to maintain skin luster and aging resistance and skin cancer:

Steps to get rid of dry skin

The strangest cosmetics in Europe

Water:

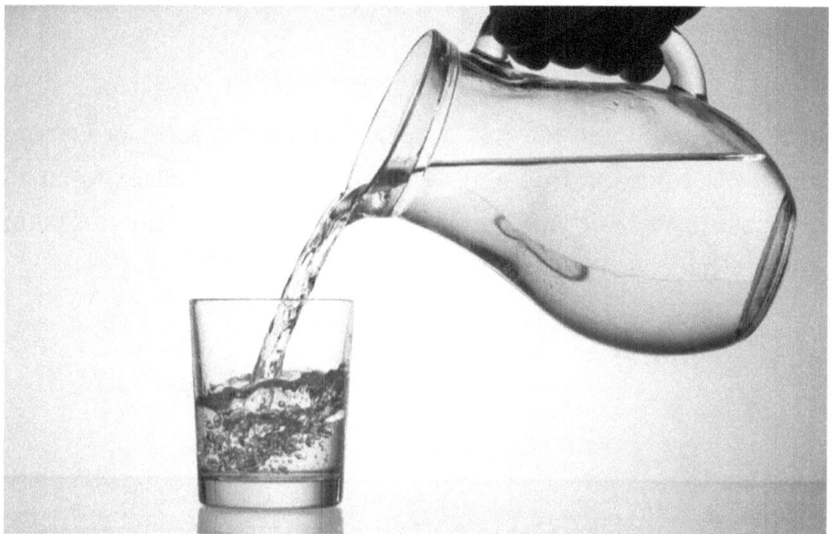

advised to eat at least two liters a day to avoid loss of fluids in the body, thus gaining vitality and vitality of the body.

Green tea:

Protects against skin cancer, and recommends taking two cups a day to get the desired benefit.

Wheat Full of beans, tuna and Brazilian almonds:

It is rich in selenium and zinc. Selenium is an antioxidant, responsible for skin elasticity and protects the skin from ultraviolet radiation. Brazilian almonds are very rich in zinc, controlling fat and some hormones that cause acne.

Salmon, walnuts and flaxseeds:

Vitamin E is rich in omega-3 and vitamin E, and is known to protect skin and reduce sunburn. Some studies have found that vitamin E treats the problems of acne and blackheads, helps to soften the skin, and reduces the dryness and appearance of wrinkles. It is recommended to eat the sauce for daily salad and a tablespoon of flaxseed is taken in the morning breakfast with breakfast cereals.

Strawberry, cranberry, red peach:

It is an antioxidant and has a very important role in protecting skin cells from damage and aging, especially when exposed to high sunlight, and may contribute to the prevention of skin cancer. Red peach is the best antioxidant.

pomegranate:

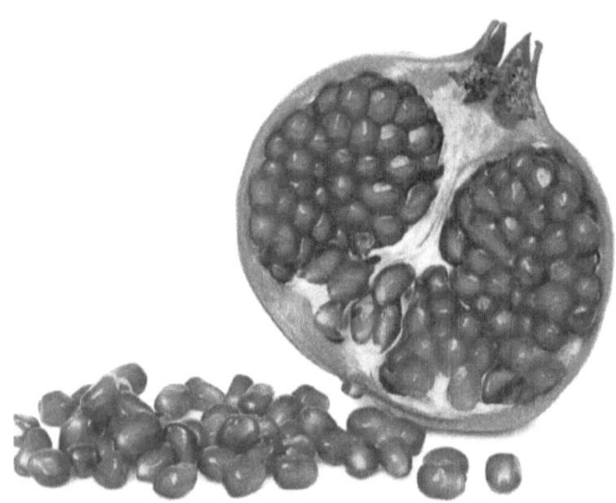

In addition to antioxidants,pomegranate helps the skin to produce the collagen necessary for the skin's freshness and protection from aging and maintain skin elasticity.

Tomato paste:

It is very rich in lycopene, an important antioxidant. Reduce cell damage and thus protect the skin from aging, and also contains vitamin C.

avocado:

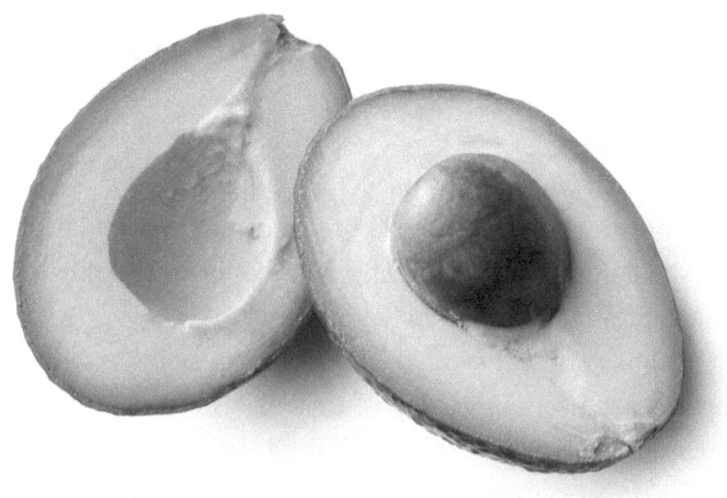

It is the best natural product for the youth of the skin because it is rich in vitamin E, and reduces the dryness of the skin and cracks is ideal for dry skin and rich in antioxidants. Adding two slides to power will produce the desired results.

cells.

Vitamin tablets can not replace fresh foods, and women are never advised to take vitamins under the pretext of keeping the skin against aging, a phenomenon that is now common among women. Taking the notes mentioned above believes that the body is better absorbed in the daily vitamins that women need.

Creams or cosmetics?

The importance of using creams in the form of different acids or vitamins; but the method of healthy nutrition is not less important in maintaining the freshness of the skin to the effect of creams. Cosmetic creams alone are not enough in the freshness of the skin and maintain its youth, because the body needs certain types of food, minerals and vitamins to remain young, and the person who does not eat the daily needs of the food referred to fall prey to aging at an early age.

Sex keeps young

A beauty touch with camel milk

Every woman who wants her skin to enjoy softness and beautiful colors should eat a diet containing iron that gives the skin a good color and prevents it from fluctuating.

There are many other tips to keep skin young, and we recommend eating at least 5 servings a day of fresh fruits and vegetables rich in vitamins, minerals, fiber and drinking water to maintain healthy skin always reflects the health of the body from the inside.

If your skin is sensitive or greasy, you should reduce your intake of strong coffee, chocolate and some spices (pepper, ginger, curry powder, sweet peppers and mustard) and fermented cheese, and try to avoid large amounts of fat and sugar

should eat low amounts of sugar and fat, increase the consumption of fresh fruits and vegetables, and also drink a little caffeine. The antioxidant foods are made up of vitamins D, C, A, iron, magnesium, copper, zinc, and other important ingredients to resist aging and those foods:

Foods that help to strengthen memory

and concentration

Strengthen memory

Strengthen the memory is not limited to the elderly, we are all in the stage of forgetting some things in a public place or forget what we read and more annoying position of forgetfulness is to meet someone you have not met him for some time and do not remember or even remember his name !! Students also sometimes suffer from poor memory, many of them are nerds and work hard and may forget the information they read and studied at the exam, the most important foods that help to strengthen memory.

Foods that help to strengthen memory:

1. Dark chocolate: Contains antioxidants that fight aging and fight memory loss

2.Tot: also contains antioxidants

3. Green Tea:

Taking a cup of green tea in the morning helps improve memory

4. Eggplant: helps the brain maintain the level of Omega 3, which enhances memory and strengthens it in addition to contain antioxidants

5. Cholesterol: Whole grains generally help reduce cholesterol in the blood and thus increase blood flow to the brain

6. Tomatoes: Also contain a high percentage of antioxidants

7. Apple: fights the substances in which Alzheimer's and forgetfulness

8. Grapes and grapes: rich in vitamin C, which helps to strengthen memory

9. Nuts: rich in omega-3, vitamin-6 and antioxidants, all of which are effective in stimulating and strengthening memory, especially nuts. It is very similar to the brain and has great benefits for memory, brain and brain health.

10. Seafood: Rich in omega-3 that activates brain cells

11. onions: especially red onions is known that onions was a cure for most diseases in ancient Egyptians

12. Citrus and citrus: Citrus contains generally vitamin C, which is known to help strengthen the brain

13. Meat, especially red: Meat of all kinds contains vitamin B12, which contributes to the strengthening of memory significantly

14. Eggs: Contains proteins and vitamins that benefit the brain and memory significantly

Sports also play an important role in strengthening memory as it reduces the proportion of fat and cholesterol in the blood and helps in blood flow to and from the heart and brain

Foods that strengthen immunity

The flu season is approaching us! Do you want to fight those diseases that take advantage of winter weather or any change in the atmosphere to attack you? Do you want to protect your body from viruses that spread in your work environment or in your children's school? If, along with attention to cleanliness should work to strengthen the immune system.

It does not mean that eating oranges, for example, will drive vitamin C to protect you from the disease.

Enhancing the immune system depends on a combination of eating healthy foods rich in vitamins and minerals throughout the year, eating meals of colored fruits and vegetables, drinking 8-10 glasses of water a day, exercising, and getting enough sleep to rest your body.

Visit your nearest neighborhood and choose a variety of ingredients to serve as an additional protective shield for your meals. Of these components:

Yogurt:

Rich in probiotics or "active organisms" that are healthy bacteria that keep the gut and intestines free of pathogenic germs. Eating one cup a day may reduce your chances of getting the flu.

citrus fruits:

The fruits of orange, grapefruit and lemon are rich in vitamin C, which is thought to increase the production of white blood cells, the key to fight inflammation. The human body does not store or produce vitamin C, so taking a daily dose of this vitamin is very important.

Broccoli:

This type of vegetable is rich in vitamins (A, C, E) and also contains a variety of antioxidants that help your body to fight infections and infections.

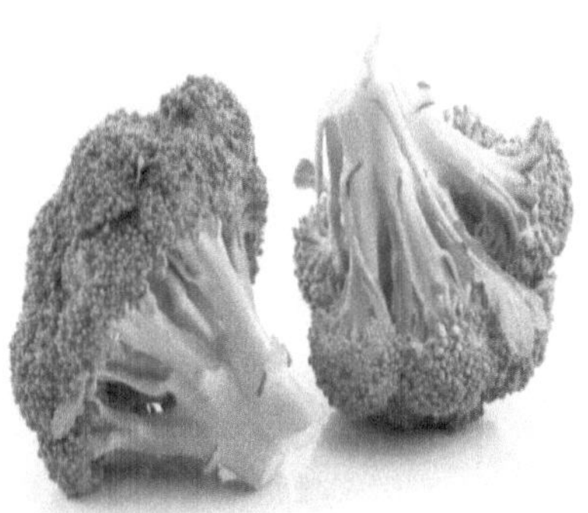

Broccoli should be cooked as little as possible to maintain beneficial nutrients.

Spinach:

These green leaves are rich not only in vitamin C but also in many antioxidants, including folic acid, which helps the body build new cells and repair DNA.

sweet potato:

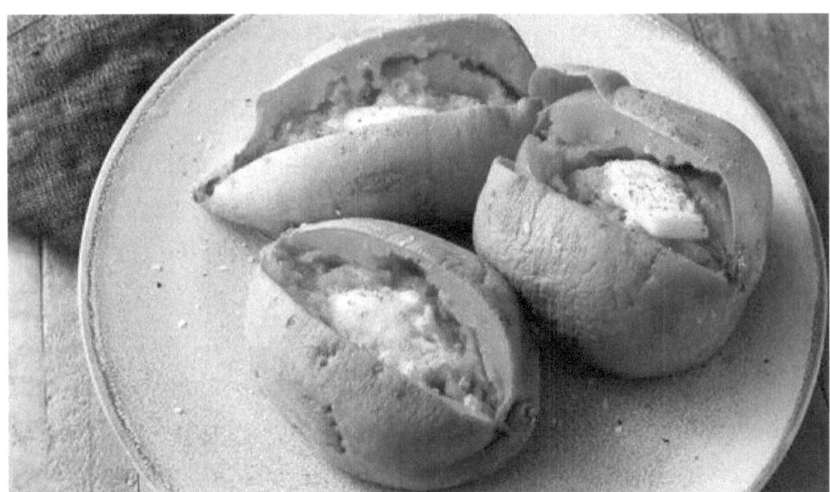

Sweet potatoes and many other vegetables such as cantaloupe, pumpkin and squash are rich in carotenoids converted into vitamin A, which contains antioxidants, and can reduce the risk of some cancers, and is associated with the fight against aging and aging.

Fish

Fish and crustaceans such as oysters, lobsters and lobsters are rich in zinc and selenium, which helps white blood cells produce certain proteins that cleanse certain viruses from your body. Fish are also rich in omega-3 fatty acids, which reduce inflammation, increase airflow and protect the lungs from colds and respiratory infections.

Fruits of berries:

The fruits of blackberries, berries, strawberries and acai berries are rich in a wide range of antioxidants that contribute to the elimination of free radicals and protect the body against inflammation.

Garlic mushroom:

The fungus is rich in selenium, B vitamins, niacin and riboflavin, which enhance your immunity and protect you from flu.

Garlic:

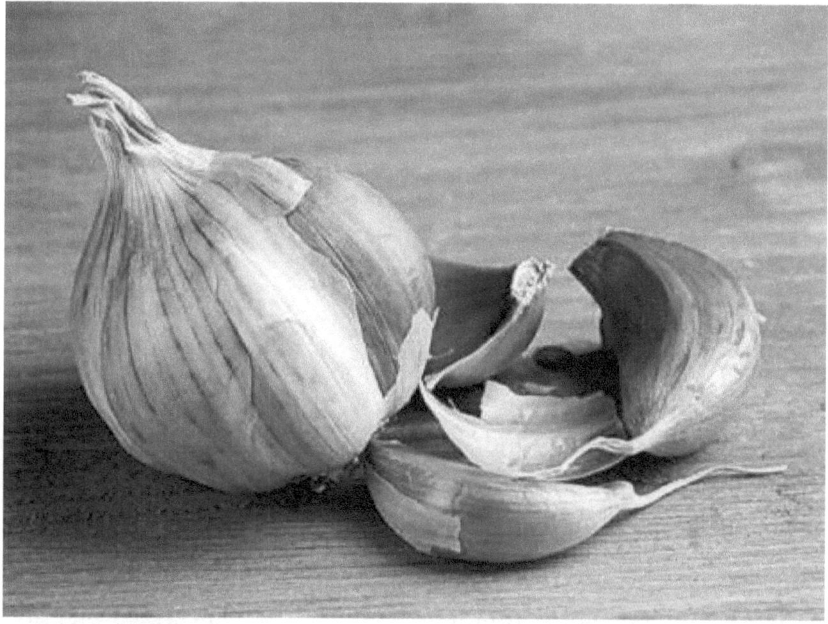

A major ingredient that is introduced into the dishes of most kitchens around the world, and the properties of enhanced immunity that is characterized by garlic from the large concentration of compounds containing sulfur.

Green tea:

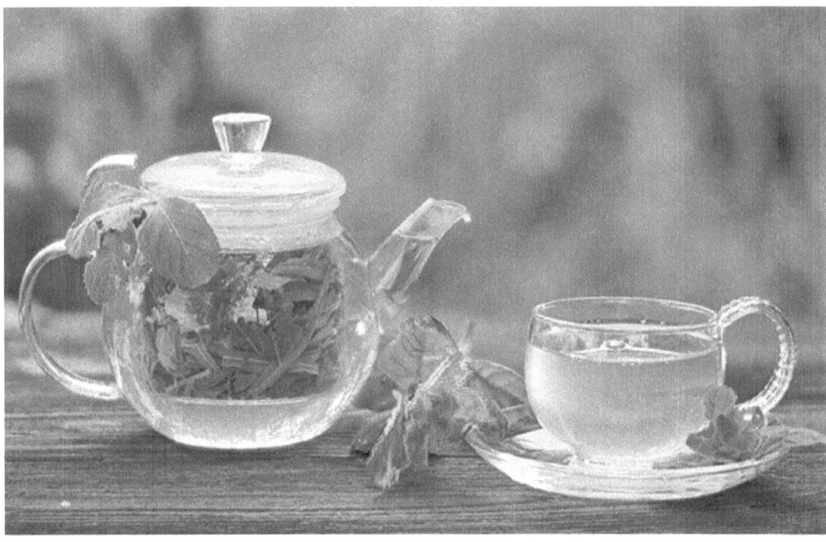

Rich in antioxidants and amino acids, which help produce immune cells that fight germs.

Plan daily meals to include a variety of fruits, vegetables, proteins, and healthy fats. Be sure to follow a healthy lifestyle to help strengthen your immune system and ensure protection against various diseases

Natural Viagra for men

 Some men suffer from erectile dysfunction, which makes them unable to perform their marital duties to the fullest. This problem affects about 80 million men around the world according to specialized studies and statistics, and may cause them grief and loss of self-confidence.

Beware of these sports .. negatively affect your ability to sex

But do not worry, erectile dysfunction does not always need to see a doctor to get rid of it. As there are natural foods with natural tonics that help the man and stimulate his desire, and give him the ability to improve his performance, we show you the most prominent of these foods after consulting a group of doctors with competence:

1 - Oysters: is a special food of love, the legend says that the famous lover Casanova, was dealing with dozens of oysters a day. The reason for this is that oysters improve the level of dopamine Dopamine, which stimulates sexual desire in both men and women. It is also rich in zinc, which makes it important for the production of testosterone hormone and ensure the health of sperm.

2. **Melon**:

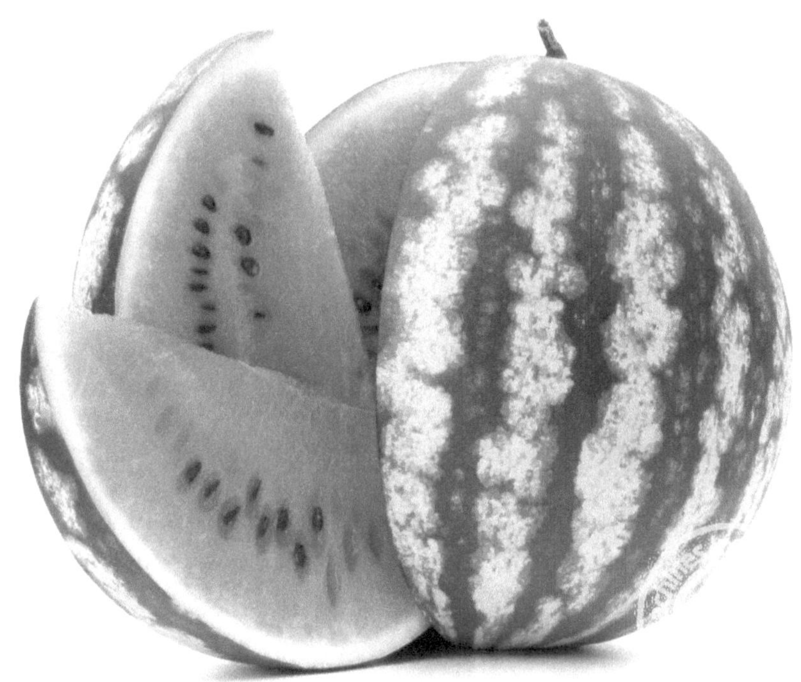

Some experts call the watermelon the new Viagra title. "Eating watermelon produces a similar effect to Viagra in whole-body blood vessels, which may increase libido," said researcher BhimuPAtil at the University of Texas. The fruit also contains citulline, which is known to be beneficial to the blood system and helps to relax blood vessels , Which increases libido.

The dilemma of the ugly "sexual face" is how it deals with it

3. Cocoa or chocolate: Chocolate comes from cocoa beans, and the Aztecs have described cocoa as the food of the gods. Today's nutritionists know that cocoa is a powerful food. It also contains phenylletamine, a stimulant that stimulates the senses of pleasure and happiness.

Maca roots are roots known in Peru as natural sex stimulants since the Inca. According to health experts, the roots of the maka are used in Peru to increase physical strength, ability to continue and extend the body energy and stimulate fertility and sexual desire.

Who are the most satisfied people about their sexuality?

Pumpkin seeds or pumpkin seeds: These seeds are rich in zinc useful in the production of sperm, and prevents the weakness of testosterone in men as well. It is also rich in vitamins and minerals that stimulate sexual desire, such as vitamin B, E, C and D, as well as vitamin K. Minerals include calcium, potassium and phosphorus. It is also rich in omega-3 fatty acids, which increase the levels of hormones that stimulate desire.

6- Celery: You may not think of celery as a stimulant for sexual desire. But according to Walter Gaman and Mark Anderson, authors of "Stay Young: 10 Sure Steps to Perfect Health." Stay Young: Ten Proven Steps to Ultimate Health. Eating celery increases the levels of pheromones in the man's sweat, making it more attractive to women.

Sudden erectile dysfunction, causes and treatment

7 - Chilies: The Capsaicin Capsaicin located in the warm, which gives him a bitter taste, is also promoting sexual desire. It increases the release of chemicals that increase the proximity and lead to the release of the hormone Andorphin, which makes you excited.

8. Figs: Legends say figs were one of Cleopatra's favorites. According to Dr. Nilini Chilkov NaliniChilkov, the fig of sensory foods. The ancient Greeks estimated figs and introduced them to gold, linking it to fertility.

9. Garlic: Eating raw garlic increases a man's sexual desire. It is the bitter taste of garlic that stimulates desire. Garlic contains allicin, which increases blood flow to sexual organs. But garlic must be consumed for a whole month, in order to reap the benefits of sex.

Pomegranate: Foods that increase energy levels in the body. Studies have shown that pomegranate juice works as a Viagra, and one cup of it makes you able to perform well. It is rich in antioxidants that help the blood to reach your sexual organs, which improves its performance.

The latter is a list
 of the longest-lived people and how many lived because the above was the outcome of their experiences in life and was the pattern of their behavior

10 - Japanese Camaro Hong, born in 1887, died in 2003 at the age of 116 years.

9. Carrie White, born in 1874, died in 1991 at the age of 116 years.

8. Elizabeth Bolden, born in 1890, died in 2006 at the age of 116 years.

7. Japanese Tyne Ikei, born in 1879, died in 1995 at the age of 116 years.

6. Ecuadorian Maria Escher DiCabovilla, born in 1889, died in 2006, 18 days before her 117th birthday.

5. Canadian Mary Miller, born in 1880, died in 1998 at the age of 117 years.

4. Lucy Hanna, born in 1875 and died in 1993 at the age of 117 years.

3. Sarah Knoss, born in 1880, died 33 hours before the age of 119 at the age of 119.

2. Shiguchio Izumi, the most famous man in the Guinness Book of Records, died at the age of 120.

1 - French Jane Calmint, is the most famous person in the Guinness Book of Records, and died at the age of 121 years e told them about his hometown, And from here I knew that area. Imagine humans 160 years old do not get sick .. Hunza tribes the most human beings the longest life on Earth.

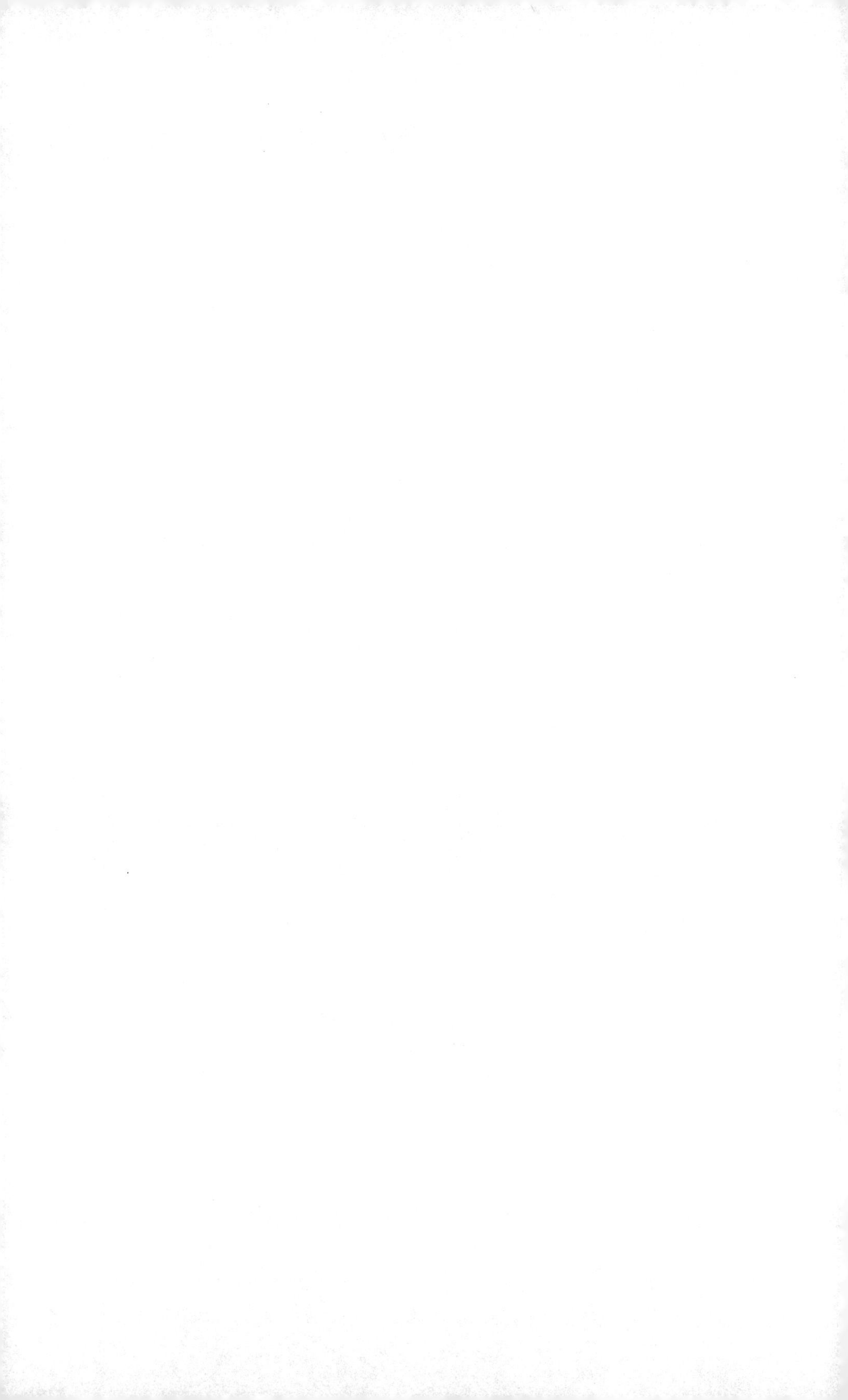

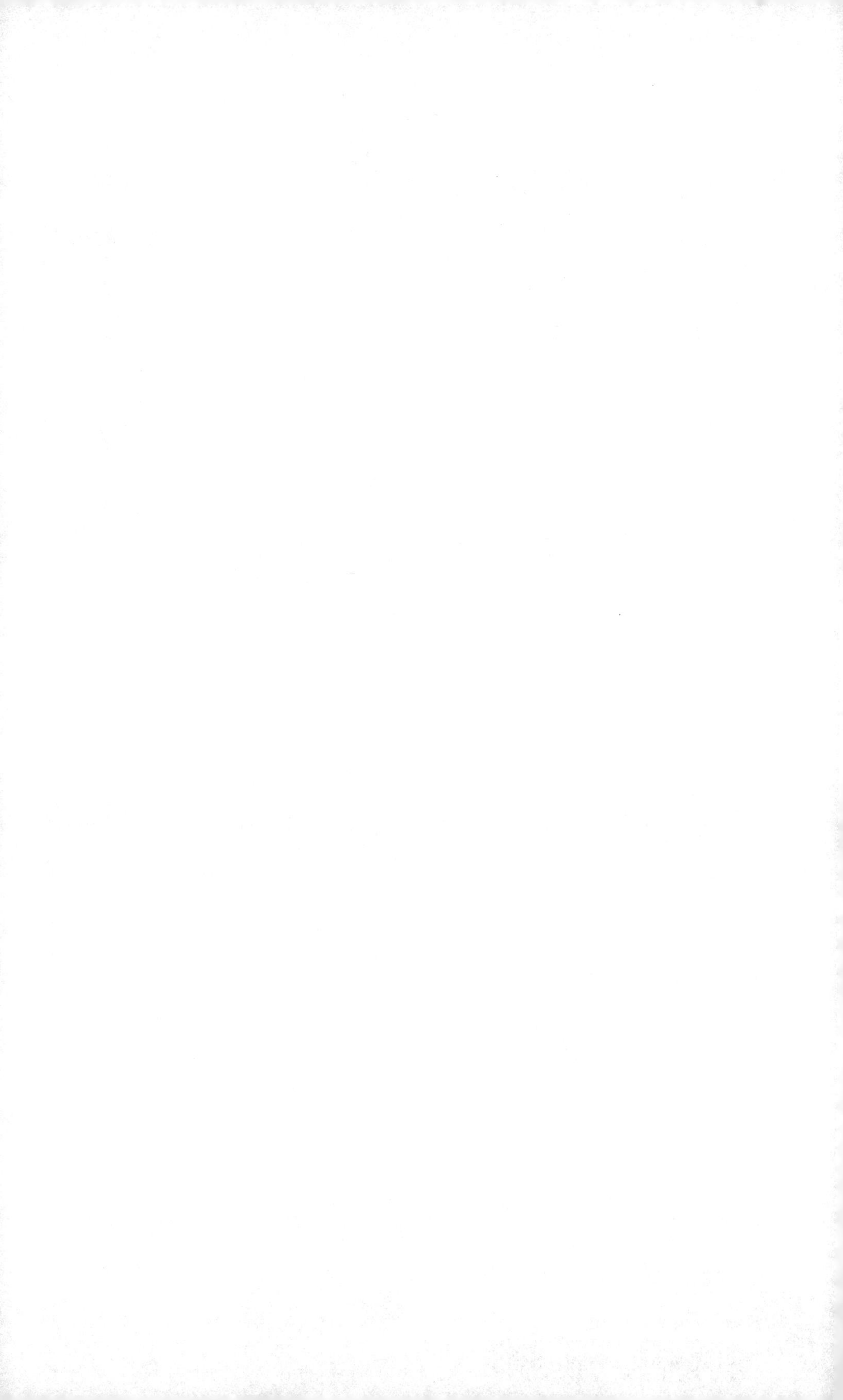